The Big Pharma Conspiracy

The Drugging of America for Fast Profits

By Max Fitzer

Copyright 2015 by Max Fitzer.

Published by Make Profits Easy LLC

Profitsdaily123@aol.com

facebook.com/MakeProfitsEasy

Table of Contents

Introduction 4

Chapter 1: The History of the Big Pharma Boom 20

Chapter 2: Mass Marketing and the Media 29

Chapter 3: Diabetes, Cancer and Alzheimer's .. 40

Chapter 4: The Drugging of Our Youth 58

Chapter 5: Conspiracy Theories 78

Chapter 6: Squelching Innovative Medical Practices 98

Chapter 7: Helpless in America 103

Conclusion 108

Introduction

Who is this big bad wolf known as Big Pharma? The name is repeatedly in the news but do you know exactly who they are? The term is a nickname bestowed upon the massive pharmaceutical companies frequently found on the Fortune 500 list. The connotation of Big Pharma is definitely a negative one. Between the conspiracy theories and the reality of billions these companies earn in profits, it is hard for an average citizen to not feel adversely towards these megalithic beasts.

Before anyone can justifiably get behind the anti-Big Pharma train, it is critical to garner as much knowledge on who they are, what they do, and why. In order to make informed decisions and not just be another sheep following the pack, it is a necessary and responsible measure to understand exactly who the "enemy" is and how they grew into the giants they are today. There are American companies as well as internationally based organizations. This book will take you through the history of the largest companies, discussing the impact they have on society, our youth, disease, and the global economy. Not only will you have an extensive understanding of who the players are, but you will also learn how to contribute to the effort to bring them under control.

Who is Big Pharma?

There are approximately 12 companies that make up Big Pharma. The six American companies are Johnson & Johnson, Pfizer, Abbott Laboratories, Merck & Co, Eli Lilly, and Bristol-Myers Squibb. Roche hails from Switzerland and Astra-Zeneca has its roots in the UK and Sweden. A familiar name may be GlaxoSmithKline, based in the UK and Bayer Healthcare from Germany. Lastly, Sanofi calls France its home. The names probably ring a bell because of the commercials you may see on television for the numerous prescription medications available for every ailment known to humankind.

Johnson & Johnson has become a household name, mostly because of its consumer products branch of the company. Incorporated in 1887, the company founded in New Brunswick, NJ by three brothers initially manufactured surgical dressings. Through the turn of the century, the company expanded into first aid kits, and most famously, baby products. In 1961, Johnson & Johnson acquired Janssen Pharmaceutica, based in Belgium. This exploded J & J into a profitable market of prescription drugs such as the anti-psychotic Risperdal and the Alzheimer's medication, Reminyl. Next, they expanded into eye care and most significantly, the development of the revolutionary coronary stent, rocketing the company into the billion dollar sales category. Currently the company has 3 main focuses: consumer products, medical devices and diagnostics, and of course, pharmaceuticals. In 2014, J & J netted over $16 billion in profit.

Pfizer, founded in 1849 by two German immigrants, Charles Pfizer and Charles F. Erhart in New York City, started out as a manufacturer of fine chemicals. The Civil War brought about the need for medicines like painkillers and antiseptics. Pfizer jumped on the opportunity and continued even after the war, splitting their focus between drugs and manufacturing citric acid for the booming soft drink industry. Though they began as a chemical manufacturer, the onset of World War II brought a demand for penicillin. Pfizer worked closely with government scientists to produce the majority of the antibiotic used on the Allied side during the entire war. This set Pfizer up for massive success in the antibiotic field. Continued research and development led to the production of well-known prescriptions such as Lipitor, Lyrica, Diflucan, Zithromax (famous Z-pack), and the ever popular Viagra. Pfizer is the largest of the Big Pharma companies, and reported a meager $9.1 billion net profit in 2014.

Abbott Laboratories, which began its illustrious history as Abbott Alkaloidal Company, was founded by a young doctor by the name of Wallace C. Abbott, a graduate of the University of Michigan in 1888. Dr. Abbott devised a product called "Dosimetric granules" from the alkaloid part of medicinal plants. It was the most accurate form of dosing medication available. In 1919, the company changed its name to Abbott Laboratories, denoting its dedication to research. Abbott Labs are well known for their breakthroughs in anesthetics, and radiopharmaceuticals leading to cutting edge thyroid treatments. Though the last several decades, the company acquisitioned many smaller companies, and most impressively spawned AbbVie in 2013, a new sister company committed to research in the global biopharmaceutical field. In 2014, they only managed to bring in $1.7 billion in net profit.

Merck & Co. was born from the oldest pharmaceutical company in the world. In 1668,

Friedrich Jacob Merck purchased Angel Pharmacy in Germany which to this day is still retained by Friedrich's descendants. The family grew the business throughout the years and in 1891 established an American subsidiary called Merck & Co. in New Jersey, while Merck in Germany became Merck KGaA. Due to World War I, Merck lost its international subsidiaries and Merck & Co. became its own independent company that we know today. Beginning as a publisher of medical reference books, today Merck is synonymous with Vioxx, a failed drug as well as Claritin and Clarinex, which were originally manufactured by Schering and Plough, now owned by Merck. Merck brought $11.92 billion in net profit for 2014.

Colonel Eli Lilly, a veteran of the Civil War, is for whom the Big Parma company is named. Disgusted with the quality of medications available to soldiers during the war, he was committed to manufacturing the highest quality pharmaceuticals. He began with only 4 employees, three of which were family. Working closely with Frederick Banting and Charles Best, the co-founders of insulin, Eli Lilly became the first manufacturer of insulin, treating the at the time deadly disease of diabetes. Lilly set his company apart from others because he was more interested in philanthropy than greed. From the Panic of 1893 to the 1906 San Francisco Earthquake up to the Lilly Endowment, Lilly gave back to the world, and helped many in need. To this day, Eli Lilly is in the top ten most philanthropic organizations in the world. In 2014, the net profits reported for Eli Lilly were $2.39 billion.

The last of the American Big Pharma companies is Bristol-Myers Squibb. As you have seen with the other American companies' pasts, their company has a long history of mergers and acquisitions. Edward R. Squibb founded his pharmaceutical company in Brooklyn, NY circa 1858. In 1887, two friends named William McLaren Bristol and John Ripley Myers invested

$5,000 into a pharmaceutical manufacturing company in Clinton, NY. The companies ran parallel to each other, both being major players in the antibiotic production boom from World War II. The two did not merge until 1989, becoming the Big Pharma goliath we know today. BMS earned $2 billion in net profit for the fiscal year 2014.

Roche, a pharmaceutical company headquartered in Switzerland, was founded by Fritz Hoffman-La Roche in 1896. By the 1914, it was an international company with offices in the US, Italy, Brazil, China and India to name just a few. Roche saw the potential for standardized medicine in the global market and capitalized on it early. War torn Europe and Russia took its toll on the company, being boycotted by Germany during World War I and losing assets in Russia during the Revolution of 1917. In the early 1930's, a resurgence of vitamin demand spurred the company to once again become prosperous. Over the years, they focused on pharmaceutical research, leading them to a diverse product portfolio from antidepressants to chemotherapy agents. They are most well-known for their tranquilizers, Valium and Rohypnol. In 2014, Roche reported approximately $9.3 billion in Swiss francs.

Two leaders in the pharmaceutical world merged in 1998 to form the colossal Astra-Zeneca. Astra AB, based out of Sweden was founded in 1913 to compete with the German based companies that dominated the market in Sweden. Zeneca, based in the UK, was formed in 1993 when Imperial Chemical Industries split up into two independent companies, one focusing on agrochemicals and the other on pharmaceuticals. Zeneca bought Salick Healthcare, a US corporation focused on cancer research and medicines, and in turn became a leader in cancer care treatments. Astra AB discovered Losec (Prilosec) and Xylocaine (lidocaine) and AstraZeneca is best known for Crestor (everyone has seen the commercials!). They reportedly earned a cool $748 million in net profit for 2014.

Perhaps the most infamous name in the Big Pharma group is GSK, or GlaxoSmithKline. Like others in this elite group, GSK has a long history, filled with mergers and acquisitions. It began in 1830 when John K. Smith opened a drugstore in Philadelphia, PA. Mahlon Kline was hired as a bookkeeper for Smith, and over the years took on more responsibilities which led to the name becoming Smith, Kline and Company. In 1859, Thomas Beecham started a laxative business in England by the name of Beecham Pills. Then in New Zealand, 1904 a Brit by the name of Joseph Nathan launches a trading company that became trademarked in 1906 as Glaxo. If all of that isn't confusing enough, there were many more mergers leading up to the 1989 merger of Beecham and Smith, Kline and Company and finally in 2000, Glaxo Wellcome mergers and the company we know today as GlaxoSmithKline is born. The broad spectrum of business avenues all the merged companies have traveled on are too long to list here however the most notable in GSK's history (separate and together) are vaccines, pharmaceuticals, and consumer healthcare products. They lay claim to Imitrex, Augmentin, Flonase, Zantac and Paxil just to name a few. In 2014, GSK pulled in $2.76 billion.

Bayer aspirin has been a household medicine cabinet staple for decades. Bayer AG is a holding company for all the subsidiaries, management and operational companies. In 1863, a partnership began in Barmen, Germany between a master dyer and a dyestuffs salesman. The salesman, Friedrich Bayer and his partner, Johann Friedrich Weskott felt there was a big opportunity in the manufacturing and sales of synthetic dyes. In 1899, having opened a research laboratory in 1878, Friedrich Bayer and Co released Bayer Aspirin, which was labeled as the drug of the century. From chemicals and explosives through the World Wars to women's contraception in 1960, Bayer has been changing with the times. Today, the company is focused on four areas of business: animal health, pharmaceuticals, consumer healthcare, and medical care. Bayer reported a net profit for 2014 of $3.43 billion.

Last, and certainly not least, is the behemoth Sanofi which is based in France. Beginning in 1718, the number of mergers and corporate takeovers that has brought us the Sanofi we know today is long and confusing. They built a successful business on manufacturing plant derivatives for the production of medication, cardiovascular therapy, cancer treatments, and most recently the production of vaccines for many infectious diseases, including influenza. In 2004, Sanofi merged with Aventis, another big player in the pharmaceutical arena and the leviathan is now known as Sanofi-Aventis. In 2014, Sanofi-Aventis earned $4.3 million euros in net income.

Why learn the history of all the Big Pharma players? It is critical to understand the small beginnings of these companies, many of which can trace their roots back over a century or more, for the purpose of seeing how the greed of our society has grown over decades. The effect these companies have had on society and even government is a formidable one. Between lawsuits, controversies and even conspiracy theories, these companies have grown so large and have such a long reach; it almost seems they are above the law.

More than 70% of Americans are on some form of prescription drugs, and more than 50% are on more than one. (CBS NEWS June 20, 2013) There are economic and psychological ramifications that almost three quarters of the country are drugged.

> A major contributor to the U.S. economy, the biopharmaceutical sector generates high-quality jobs and powers economic output for the U.S. economy, serving as

the "the foundation upon which one of the United States' most dynamic innovation and business ecosystems is built," according to the Battelle Technology Partnership Practice. (The Economic Impact of the Pharmaceutical Industry – PhRMA)

The success of the pharmaceutical industry represents hundreds of thousands of jobs, not to mention billions of dollars pumped into the economy in the form of tax revenues, individual income, and discretionary spending money. Pharmaceutical companies pump about $500 billion into research and development (R&D). These funds go to supply vendors, schools and institutions, and of course, the employees of the R&D sector. Battelle has researched the economic impact on 33 states across the country, and in Massachusetts alone, the biopharmaceutical industry represents $38 billion in economic output. This includes everything from direct output such as jobs from administration to management to transportation and indirect output like IT support and real estate/construction companies. The foundation of our economy is literally resting on Big Pharma's success. If the pharmaceutical industry were to fail for any reason, it would mean an economic disaster of epic proportions.

The psychological impact is another can of worms that has just begun to open.

> "One in four women in their 40's and 50's is taking antidepressants. Though the US contains just 5% of the world population, it consumes over half of all prescribed medication and a phenomenal 80% of the world's supply of painkillers."

Our society is riddled with drugs. The quantity of illegal drugs consumed by Americans yearly does not even come close to the amount of prescription medications. Between kids with pills for ADHD and ADD to anyone and everyone on some form of painkillers, the effects are staggering. We are drugging ourselves into a coma; becoming a culture of good sheep that follow the shepherd, in this case Big Pharma. And what does Big Pharma do? Gets greedier and greedier and their wallets grow fatter and fatter. While the top pharmaceutical companies only represent about 4% of the Fortune 500, the profit they bring in combined is more than the top 10 companies earn combined. The profit margins are wide, and the market share is deep for Big Pharma.

How did this industry get started? When did it turn from helping to hurting people?

Chapter 1: The History of the Big Pharma Boom

As discussed in the introduction, Big Pharma has roots that go deep. Even though the companies we know today are a result of mergers, take-overs, acquisitions, and demergers, many are still over 100 years old. Beginning with botanical extracts and vitamins through to synthetic medications, these companies have traveled a long and profitable road.

The boom really started for Big Pharma in World War II, however looking at World War I can help us understand the gradual shift to greed. As discussed, Bayer began as a dye manufacturer, dealing with organic chemicals and processes. It is not difficult to see the jump from that to chemical warfare. This was one opportunity pharmaceutical companies saw to turn a profit during the war. Bayer even went so far as to build a School of Chemical Warfare. The chemical branch of Bayer went on to merge into Germany's single largest pharmaceutical company known as IG Farben, who in turn was the biggest donor to Hitler's campaign. What is the most impactful event from World War I is war torn Germany's inability to distribute pharmaceuticals worldwide. This spurred production in the UK, France and the United States, uncontested by the German super power IG Farben and Bayer.

These events lead us to World War II, the war that spawned the Greatest Generation. Medical breakthroughs were happening at a rapid rate. The discovery of penicillin was ground breaking. Eli Lilly had founded a pure method manufacturing of insulin to help control diabetes, which was a killer disease before this finding. Streptomycin was discovered as an effective treatment for tuberculosis in 1943 by Merck.

When Alexander Fleming realized the properties of penicillium's mold, a huge collaboration began to manufacture and mass produce penicillin. This goal was achieved in World War II and many soldiers have Big Pharma to thank for their lives. Without it, the death tolls could have been doubled.

The darker side of World War II presents us with IG Farben's nefarious plan to take over the pharmaceutical world.

> "In each and every country Hitler's Wehrmacht invaded, the first act was to rob the chemical, petrochemical and pharmaceutical industries and assign them – free of charge – to the I.G. Farben empire."

The test products devised by IG Farben were used in the concentration camps, essentially pharmaceutical labs for the German conglomerate. This is what padding an election fund earns you: free reign to do whatever you want. Between Farben and the US pharma cartel, money was made hand over fist during World War II. The lessons learned in these years would serve them well in the future, such as mass production and distribution on a large scale. The pharmaceutical giants had come a long way from the meager beginnings of small apothecaries and chemical manufacturers.

During the ensuing years, business was good. The discovery and manufacturing of the birth control pill, more effective treatments for cancer, diabetes, and anti-infective medications kept the pharmaceutical companies on a steady flow of income. The death rate in the post-World War II era declined from 2% to 6%, owing to the number of vaccines and anti-infectious treatments that were produced in that time. The polio vaccine was founded in 1952 by Jonas Salk. Merck had a significant impact on vaccinations, such as rubella (1969), measles (1962), and mumps (1967). By the time the 1970's rolled around, cellular and molecular biology were combining with pharmaceutical research which gave birth to the biotechnology age.

If Big Pharma felt they had made a good run up to this point, they had no idea what newly elected President Reagan had in store for them.

Reagan's policies were very pro-business. This created a shift not only in government policy, but in society as well. Before 1980, the American way of life of working hard, making a decent living was well respected. Absurd wealth was not. The subtle shift of the American people began at this juncture, where wealth began to be revered. It was a status symbol to achieve. Big Pharma leapt on it and became a beacon of affluence in the 80's. Reagan's presidency marked the first rift in the gap between the rich and poor, one that continues to grow to this very day.

Biotechnology was a raging machine, waiting to be unleashed. Two major policies literally unleashed the beast.

The Bayh-Dole Act of 1980, signed by Carter just before Reagan took office, states:

> "It is the policy and objective of the Congress to use the patent system to promote the utilization of inventions arising from federally supported research

or development; to encourage maximum participation of small business firms in federally supported research and development efforts; to promote collaboration between commercial concerns and nonprofit organizations, including universities; to ensure that inventions made by nonprofit organizations and small business firms are used in a manner to promote free competition and enterprise; to promote the commercialization and public availability of inventions made in the United States by United States industry and labor; to ensure that the Government obtains sufficient rights in federally supported inventions to meet the needs of the Government and protect the public against nonuse or unreasonable use of inventions; and to minimize the costs of administering policies in this area."

Translation? The cost of research is an exorbitant one. The act allowed universities and small businesses, who receive government funding, to patent their research, and then grant exclusivity to the drug company for manufacturing and marketing. By patenting it, the universities and small businesses earn royalties and make money also. Prior to this, those in the field of academia were not the abundant earners they have become in the 21st century. It was a win-win situation all around because everyone makes money! With 100+ years of experience and perseverance, Big Pharma was hitting the big time. All the knowledge of mass production and distribution they gained from the 1800's on could now be put to a lucrative use, without having to rely on their own scientists for discoveries.

The second act that impacted the pharmaceutical industry was the Hatch-Waxman Act. The law was formally known as Drug Price Competition and Patent Term Restoration Act of 1984.

Simply, it gives a monopoly to the drug companies on name brand drugs. They can exclusively market their patent for an extended period of time, and when the time runs out other companies can produce copies of the drug, known as generic drugs. The implementation of this policy skyrocketed the drug companies into a whole new stratosphere of revenues and profit. Marketing became the name of the game and pushing their drugs into mainstream America.

In 1986, Reagan signed the Federal Technology Transfer Act, allowing government agencies to collaborate with the private sector, i.e. Big Pharma, and essentially turn profits by selling the research to drug companies, though only 5% of their annual budget. This was a defining moment because it truly begins the close relationship between the pharmaceutical industry and the US government.

With all of these policies written into law during the 1980's, Big Pharma went from a solid, stable business to a booming giant. The industry had lulled society into a comfortable and trusting mentality, having done so much good throughout history in saving lives, extending life expectancy, and curing deadly diseases. Factor in the effortless capability to buy research from so many talented researchers and scientists in academia and the government allowed them to shift their focus to marketing, getting America hooked on drugs.

Chapter 2: Mass Marketing and the Media

Big Pharma has big reach, and fingers in many pies. They have a heavy influence on the media, and they don't even own a single radio station. Money talks and for the pharmaceutical industry, big money means big power. This includes control over the programming of the American "sheeple".

Publication bias is defined as a tendency to publish research findings that trend in the direction of the preferred result, usually a positive one. The result is that most treatments tend to be less effective in practice than the research suggests. It is staggering to know that only half of all trial results are made public or worse that positive findings are twice as likely to be published as null results. This is a common practice of the pharmaceutical research companies to skew the American public on the effectiveness of new medications.

In any published trial, there is a press release, especially if it is a history-in-the-making kind of discovery. The press release is written by the pharmaceutical company or a representative that funded, conducted, and likely patented the new drug. Because the media is under immense pressure to report the news in an instant, often they just copy the press release. This is known as parroting. Just like the bird mimics everything you say, the media regurgitates what Big Pharma says is important for the American public to know.

Every American who does not blindly follow the mainstream media knows that they are certainly lacking in the integrity department. Surprisingly, there are only 6 media mastodons left who control 95% of what you watch, read and hear daily. This is not unlike the Big Pharma cartel, perhaps why they make such nice bedfellows. In 2012, Big Pharma spent over $90 billion in advertising. Since the media has been losing ad money to the Internet, they rely heavily on the business from the pharmaceutical marketing campaigns.

Back in 2010, the media hopped on the release of a study that declared calcium supplements cause heart attacks. Add a sprinkle of sensationalism, scary headline and boom! America buys into it. The study was done with a small sample group; the doses of calcium were given with none of its beneficial co-vitamins such as magnesium, vitamin K, or omega-3 fatty acids. It is actually a well-known fact in the science and medical community that calcium can cause heart disease, when taken alone.

In December 2013, the Annals of Internal Medicine, controlled by the American Medical Association which had close ties with Big Pharma, released an opinion piece that detailed how dietary supplements are a waste of money and useless. Of course, the study they based this finding on used low dose, cheap supplements produced by Big Pharma. No mention was made in the release that using reputable dietary supplements in combination with a healthy diet and exercise will net you ideal results.

Only recently have Americans become a touch wiser in trusting the media. In a Gallup poll conducted in September of 2014, only 40% of Americans had confidence in the mass media. This is an all time, historical low though it has been trending downward for years. Still, 40% of Americans roughly translates to 120 million people. It is unknown how many of the 60% believe part of what they read, see or hear. Every day on social media sites, people share false claims and reports, covering everything from politics to health topics. These articles often go "viral" and create a stir among social media users. While most are seemingly harmless, it makes you wonder how many people believe these stories and perpetuating the sheep mentality of America.

The average American adult watches approximately 33 hours of television per week according to Nielsen data from March 2014. For five hours per day, adults are bombarded with television commercials. Depending on the programs you are watching, it is safe to say every American adult has seen a minimum of two commercials about a new drug that can help you feel younger, reduce pain, live longer, and have a great sex life. Whether for fibromyalgia, arthritis, allergies, bladder control, or depression, these commercials depict smiling, beautiful people enjoying life on sunny, warm days. Wouldn't everyone want to feel that good? Consciously we may say "this is ridiculous" however our subconscious retains this flood of information and we are literally programmed to know that one little pill can make us feel better.

Have you ever listened to the list of side effects of a miracle drug advertised on television? Prozac, also known as fluoxetine, is the most popularly prescribed antidepressant in the US, with 1 out of every 10 Americans taking it. The list of side effects for just this one drug is long and frightening. As they say in the commercials, side effects may include nervousness, nausea, dry mouth, sore throat, drowsiness, weakness, uncontrollable shaking of a part of the body, loss of appetite, weight loss, changes in sex drive or ability, excessive sweating, and suicidal thoughts. Are you kidding me? I would rather deal with the depression! There are people struggling with real clinical depression, who cannot get out of it without the help of medication. However, it is irresponsible to be unaware of how these legal drugs can affect you and should be used as a measure in conjunction with other remedies such as therapy and holistic methods.

Abilify, a drug used to treat depression and bipolar disorder, has "coma or death" as a side effect. Alli, a weight loss aid, causes bowel movements that may be uncontrollable. Veramyst, a nasal spray for allergies, can cause glaucoma and cataracts. Advair, an inhaler for asthma, can cause "asthma related death". These are just a few drugs of a VERY long list. Doctors, being led by Big Pharma, are prescribing pills for every single ailment, sniffle, and ache. Americans blindly trust the very doctors prescribing these drugs, desperate to feel as good as the people they see in the commercials.

Why have these doctors and healthcare professionals become nothing but highly paid drug dealers? Big Pharma, with their deep pockets, offer many benefits to doctors for prescribing their exclusive name brand drug of the month. The role of the pharmaceutical sales representative was initially to keep doctors informed of new products and information on drug trials and tests that they would normally be too busy to read up on themselves. Once the policies of the 80's were put into place, the pharmaceutical companies turned their focus on getting their drugs out to the general public. Whether big or small, new or old, these companies began compensating the sales reps through incentives, with small if any base salary. A shrewd sales rep knows in order to make money, you need to get the doctor to buy into the benefits of the drug in order to get the prescriptions and will use any means necessary. Not a day goes by in a doctor's office when a rep doesn't stop by with samples, promotional items, and brochures for the waiting room to dole out. Catered lunches are a common practice, delivered straight to the hospital or office. Then there are the all expenses paid conference trips, in tropical locations with luxury accommodations. Sales reps will do anything; even toe the legal and ethical lines to make their commission. Is it wrong? It is their job.

Gwen Olsen, author of *Confessions of an Rx Drug Pusher,* aired the dirty laundry of Big Pharma and how they motivate their doctors to prescribe their medications. She writes "We are trained to misinform," basically pointing the finger at Big Pharma. She alleges that when a new drug is released, not only do the sales reps minimize the side effects to the doctor, but the reps aren't even aware of 50% of the side effects. These tactics are under the directive of Big

Pharma, all in the name of making money. Even worse, Olsen talks about psychiatrists and their penchant for prescribing teens mind altering medications, without really having enough facts to properly diagnose these kids. Unlike medical doctors, or even veterinarians, psychiatrists do not need blood or urine tests. They hear a list of symptoms and slap a label on it, like ADD or ADHD. Fifteen percent of today's youth has been diagnosed with ADD or ADHD, yet only about 5% are true actual cases. Parents bring their kids in because of behavioral problems, looking for a cure or at least a reason why Johnny or Sally act up. Heaven forbid it could actually be the parent's fault.

What sales reps do could be considered out and out bribery. Some doctors may feel squeamish at the methods in which the sales reps use, but still do not do anything to stop it. In order for change to happen, it must come from the top. Big Pharma needs an overhaul on their sales practices but it is doubtful we will see a fast solution. GSK announced some changes in how their reps earn their keep, and shifting their focus more on patient improvement than number of prescriptions sold. They will also "take steps to end direct payments to health care professionals for speaking engagements as well as attendance at medical conferences." By making these changes, they are essentially admitting guilt that the practices in place are unethical at the least. While this isn't going to change the fact that there will still be benefits to doctors who prescribe GSK's drugs, it is a step in the right direction and offers hope that the rest of Big Pharma will follow suit.

In the Affordable Care Act, also known as Obamacare, a provision was made called the Sunshine Act which requires all pharmaceutical companies to disclose how much money they give to doctors in kickbacks. It is illegal to pay doctors to write subscriptions for their drugs; however it is perfectly legal for physicians to accept kickbacks for promoting their medications. In 2013, between August and December, pharmaceutical companies paid out $3.5 BILLION to 546,000 physicians and about 1,360 teaching hospitals. The largest category the money went to was for royalties, approximately $302 million. As mentioned earlier, once the Bayh-Dole Act passed, Big Pharma had gained a whole host of research resources from which they could cherry pick their next big drug. The next category was promotional speaking, $202 million. Of course, travel may occur for a conference in which a doctor speaks on behalf of a pharmaceutical company and all costs are covered, including meals and entertainment. How can we trust our doctors, knowing they are "on the take" from the very pharmaceutical companies pushing drugs for profit?

Chapter 3: Diabetes, Cancer and Alzheimer's

The big three diseases that appear to be incurable are diabetes, cancer, and Alzheimer's. These life threatening maladies represent a large chunk of the medical research, drug breakthroughs and in turn, profits for Big Pharma. There are treatments for all three of these conditions, and diabetes is now more manageable than ever however cancer and Alzheimer's are still killers today.

Diabetes has been around since ancient times. The name diabetes mellitus dates back to 250 BC, called this for the excess sugar found in urine and blood. It wasn't until 1889 when Joseph von Mering and Oskar Minkowski discovered the role of the pancreas by removing them from dogs and noting they showed all the symptoms of diabetes. In 1910, Sir Edward Albert Sharpey-Shafer discovered how the lack of insulin contributes to diabetes, coining the name insulin from "insula" meaning island. In diabetics, they are missing the islets of Langerhans in the pancreas which is the key to producing insulin.

In 1921, Banting and Best discovered a process of purifying insulin to help manage diabetes. Eli Lilly began mass producing it, essentially preventing a death sentence for those with the disease. In 1936, Sir Harold Percival Himsworth uncovered the difference between Type I and Type II diabetes, thereby improving the treatment for each type. In 1982, the first biosynthetic insulin was mass produced by using recombinant DNA, again by Eli Lilly.

Today, the tops selling drugs for treatment of diabetes rake in billions of dollars for Big Pharma. Lanlus, an insulin pen patented by Sanofi, brought in $7.6 billion last year. Interestingly, Sanofi has raised the price by 106% since 2007. This is a common practice of the pharmaceutical industry, to maximize revenues while they still hold exclusive rights to the patent.

Januvia, another top selling drug to help manage diabetes, is bringing in $4 billion in revenue to Merck. Speaking of side effects, there is a study that linked Januvia to pancreatitis however US regulators state that they have not reached a final conclusion as to what effects Januvia has on patients.

Eli Lilly continues with their focus on diabetes treatment with their drug Humalog. An injection fluid that is very popular generates $2.6 billion in revenue. Since 2007, Eli Lilly has raised the price by 111% on the prescription drug. Seeing a trend here?

Diabetes represents huge profits for Big Pharma, as there is no cure for diabetes. It has to be managed with prescription drugs. Or does it? Over 90% of patients who suffer from Type I diabetes can easily cure themselves with lifestyle changes. Type I can be eradicated with daily exercise, cutting sugar intake, increasing water consumption and quitting smoking and drinking. Sadly, most Americans are not willing to make these sacrifices when there is a pill that they can take instead. Just another example of how Big Pharma has lulled us into a society of sheep who know there is a drug to fix every problem.

Even if you did not want to change your lifestyle in order to cure yourself, there are doctors and professors working diligently to come up with cures for every ailment, including diabetes. Professor Irving Weissman discovered a cure for Type I diabetes by using adult stem cells. Shockingly, no pharmaceutical company would sponsor the clinical trials in order to get the approval for treatment to the masses. A cure for diabetes would mean billions in lost revenue for several Big Pharma companies. There isn't much they won't do to protect their fat wallets, including denying Americans a cure for Type I diabetes.

Karkinos, the Greek word Hippocrates used to describe carcinoma tumors in ancient Greece, can be traced back even earlier to 1600 BC. Bone cancer was found in mummies preserved in

Egypt. Theories about cancer have run rampant ever since. Ancient Egyptians thought cancer was caused by angering the Gods. Hippocrates thought cancer was caused by an excess of black bile in the body. Trauma theory, the thought that all cancer was caused by physical trauma to the body was disproved in the 1920's. The parasite theory was the idea that parasites which invade the human body caused cancer. It wasn't until the mid-20th century when Watson and Crick won the Nobel Prize for discovering and naming the DNA helical structure that cancer could be truly understood. Their work led scientists to understanding how genes worked, and how they were damaged by mutations.

During the 1970's, oncogenes were found to cause normal genes to grow out of control and lead to cancerous cells. Normal cells which had been damaged by viruses or exposure to carcinogens would die, however cancer cells with damaged DNA would grow and spread. By understanding how cancer grew and spread, scientists could focus on treatment and a cure.

There is a controversial story from the 1920's-30's that truly casts a dark shadow on Big Pharma, portending the future. An inventor named Royal Rife was able to isolate the human cancer virus with a high powered microscope. He cultured the sample and injected it into rats. By using an electromagnetic energy frequency on the rats, he was able to eradicate the disease. The device he created was known as the Rife Machine. In 1934, the University of Southern California heard about his work and assembled a special medical research committee to observe and study his device. Sixteen terminally ill cancer patients were brought from Pasadena hospital to be treated at Rife's lab located in San Diego. After 3 months of treatment, 14 of the 16 patients were completely cancer free. The remaining two were treated for another month, with some adjustments made on the frequency. The special committee found the cancer had been eradicated from the final two patients with the adjustments. His work was gaining notoriety, and Dr. Millbank Johnson held a banquet in honor of Rife and his work, with many renowned researchers, scientists, and doctors in attendance.

Here is where the story takes a twist, and to report only the facts will allow you to draw your own conclusions. On the night Dr. Johnson was going to release Rife's findings, he was fatally poisoned, and mysteriously all his notes and papers went missing. By 1939, anyone who had been involved in the study, and had seen the device at work denied ever meeting Rife. Rife's lab was destroyed in an arson fire. Dr. Nemes who had been replicating Rife's work was killed in a fire and all his information destroyed. Burnett Lab, where the validation of Rife's work was in progress, was also obliterated in a fire. In 1971, Rife died by an accidental lethal dose of Valium and alcohol at Grossmont Hospital.

By the 1950's, the use of electromagnetic energy to cure cancer was considered quack medicine. Rife's story became a conspiracy theory, where Rife himself said his work was sabotaged by the American Medical Association. A book published in 1987 titled *Cancer Cure That Worked* by Barry Lynes, detailing Rife's discovery and the ensuing destruction of everything and almost everyone related to it, was completely discredited by the AMA saying it was written as conspiracy theory propaganda.

Today, Rife Machines are still available, though the selling of one can be considered a felony health fraud. The AMA says his work cannot be replicated by an independent study, which means it is bogus. Conversely, on www.cancer.org, the American Cancer Society's page, you can find a section on electromagnetic energy treatment, including mention of Rife and his work. There is proof the body contains electromagnetic energy, by the use of EEG and EKG tests. Why hasn't anyone explored this field for cancer treatment? With all the medical advancements in the world, not one person has been able to get a study sponsored by any medical companies to further understand how this treatment could benefit millions. Why? Because it would cure the very disease that represents more than one quarter of the entire industry's revenue stream.

Roche is the leading cancer research and development drug company. In 2013, they garnered a staggering $25.4 billion in oncology drug sales, which is more than the other top six companies *combined*. MabThera/Rituxan, a drug that treats non-Hodgkin's lymphoma, represented $8.1 billion in revenue alone. When researching the top cancer drugs, there was an interesting fact that surfaced.

As mentioned, Rituxan is the top cancer treating drug, going from $3 billion in sales in 2011 to $25.4 billion in 2013. Listed on the Mayo Clinic's website are the side effects of this Rituxan drug; 52 common side effects, 26 less common, and an additional 18 side effects after you stop treatment. Avastin, the second leading drug only managed $2.66 billion in 2011. Lastly, Herceptin brought in $1.6 billion in revenue. What do these three drugs have in common? The patents are all owned by a company Genentech. But that's not one of the Big Pharma's we have discussed, you say? Genentech became a subsidiary of Roche in 2009. Again, it is the top 12 companies that own EVERYTHING related to the pharmaceutical industry.

New discoveries are happening every day. Why can't we cure cancer? For starters, it is widely understood that it will take more than just one miracle drug to cure cancer because cancer cells mutate so rapidly. Similar to HIV patients, a cocktail of several drugs may be needed to control and cure cancer. The problem rests in drug patents, and generic medications. Big Pharma won't collaborate or fund research that works with generic drugs because there is no profit in them. Also, where there are several companies who have different drugs to treat cancer, they won't cross the patent line because again, it may mean less revenue and who would actually own the patent? The Journal of Clinical Oncology published in 2013 that a drug called metformin, used to treat diabetes, can lead to a reduced risk of prostate cancer. Big Pharma won't sponsor any study to explore metformin either alone or in conjunction with other medications because it is a generic drug. No money.

Not to mention, often the studies that are published are so biased in favor of the pharmaceutical companies. The researchers, being funded by Big Pharma, will publish results skewing information to benefit their sponsors. The studies are rampant with false information, such as survival rates, and even effectiveness of the drug.

> "Scientists from Bayer had little luck with their studies as well. In 2011, in a paper

"Believe it or not", Bayer admitted that researchers couldn't get the same results in clinical trials on stage two of their testings. The head of Target Discovery at Bayer Schering Pharma admitted that research teams couldn't replicate the initial results of most of Bayer's studies, no matter how hard they tried. Out of 47 potential new anti-cancer drugs less than one-quarter got past stage two. The scandal that followed put an end to all anti-cancer studies at Bayer." (http://www.globalresearch.ca)

All Big Pharma wants is to make money. The only way to do that is to have sick people who stay sick, but don't die until they have purchased overpriced medication over the course of years. Keep them alive long enough to turn a profit. Make sure you don't cure them or else your cash cow will dry up.

In 1906, Dr. Alois Alzheimer performed an autopsy on a woman who presented with an unknown mental illness five years prior. The symptoms were memory loss, difficulty with language and unpredictable behavior. Her brain showed abnormalities that had not been seen before in the medical community. There were abnormal clumps and tangled bundles of fibers in her brain. These are two of the three classic signs of Alzheimer's, the third being a break in the connection of the neurons.

Even now, scientists and researchers do not know what causes Alzheimer's; however it is a definite decline in brain functions leading eventually to death. From the time of diagnosis, the disease will often take between three to nine years before it culminates in death. Memory loss is the first symptom, which can happen in non-Alzheimer patients as they age. The chance of having Alzheimer's increase drastically over 65, but can affect people as young as 40-45. The deadliest of the big three, there is no treatment to stop or reverse the effects of the disease.

The progression of the disease is a painful one for families. Watching your beloved mother, father, uncle, or aunt slowly deteriorate over years takes a toll emotionally and psychologically. Often the family is burdened with caring for the patient, whether physically or financially. Beginning with the memory loss, other symptoms include problems with language, forgetting words leading to simple vocabulary, losing capability to communicate clearly. Often patients pull away from family members and friends, slowly stop taking care of themselves, and require round the clock care. Mood swings and aggression are often signs of moderate Alzheimer's along with sundowning, named for the time of day it usually affects patients. It causes the patient to get confused and restless, often getting memories, people and things mixed up. The final stages where patients lose the ability to speak, and rely on caregivers completely becomes a waiting game for families.

As stated, no definitive known cause has been identified by scientists for Alzheimer's however, there are three common theories. Factors that can cause Alzheimer's could be genetic, environmental, lifestyle or a combination of the three. What we do know is that the brain slowly deteriorates over time, brain cells dying and there for less connectivity, causing the brain to shrink. Plaques build up in the brain made up of proteins called beta-amyloid, or amyloids for short. The tangles of protein called tau get caught up and twist, allowing a decline or stoppage of communication between neurons. There is the amyloid theory basically is the thought that massive build-up of proteins causes the brain function to slow and eventually stop. The tau theory is the main cause of Alzheimer's is the tangles of tau protein preventing communication between neurons, thereby killing brain cells.

There are only 5 FDA approved drug treatments for Alzheimer's. Three of which are cholinesterase inhibitors, supporting the amyloid theory of treatment. Pfizer manufactures Aricept, also known as Donezpil in its generic form. Janssen, a subsidiary of Johnson & Johnson has the patent on Razadyne, now available as Galantamine, the generic name. Cognex, a drug that is rarely ever prescribed because of the potential for liver failure, was patented by Warner-Lambert who merged with Pfizer in 2000. Lastly, Novartis, new to the pharmaceutical scene in 1996, has the trademark on Exelon.

The most popular, and arguably the most effective drug is Namenda or Mematine, patented by a Dublin based pharmaceutical company known as Actavis Plc. It improves memory, attention, reason, and language. It helps regulate abnormal activity of glutamate, an important chemical in the brain to help learning processes.

These patients and their families are easy prey for drug companies. No one wants to watch someone they love slowly decline, waiting for the disease to take their lives. Big Pharma makes billions a year on Alzheimer medications. It makes it a tough pill to swallow when hearing about the court appeal by Actavis made in April 2015.

In December of 2014, district superior court ruled that Actavis had to continue to offer their Alzheimer drug, Namenda IR even though they had developed a newer and recently patented version known as Namenda XR. They are the EXACT SAME DRUG, the only difference is XR is a once a day pill, whereas IR is a twice a day. Actavis' argument was that if they could not discontinue Namenda IR, when the patent runs out in 2015, it will open up the competition to make generic versions. This means they would stand to lose approximately $200 million in sales. Let's break that down: the company wants to discontinue the production of a drug because they have a new version, recently patented that they can make more money on because it is slightly different by being a time released dose. They can also charge more for the drug that is protected by patent, as it would be the only version available. Greed at its finest.

Between these three diseases alone, the pharmaceutical companies earn billions upon billions of dollars every year. These billions come from American citizen's pockets in the form of co-pays, insurance payments, and prescription fees. Diabetes patients are paying out the nose to just maintain decent health while at the very least Type I can be cured with better life choices. Though caught up in conspiracy theory, the fact that Rife's work was lost and never picked up or researched again is sinful. In essence, when Actavis went to court pleading not to continue production of Namenda IR, they were pleading to take more of your money. When is it enough?

Chapter 4: The Drugging of Our Youth

While it is nauseating how Big Pharma is bleeding the bank accounts of the sick, elderly, and grown sheeple of America, it does not even compare to what it is doing to our youth. Parents today are faced with many challenges that did not exist when their parents were raising them. In order for a middle class family to own a home, two cars, keep food on the table, and a family vacation every year, it requires both parents have full time jobs, with above average pay. Spare time is limited between shuttling kids to activities or sports practice, grocery runs, cooking dinner, keeping up with the yard and the home. When your child is unwell, either physically or mentally, it is a dangerous juggling game of doctor appointments, treatments, research and all the while maintaining balance with work. In the current climate, kids are brought to the doctor or the psychiatrist and invariably leave with a prescription. Big Pharma is literally drugging our youth.

ADHD/ADD is the most commonly diagnosed disorder in children. ADHD stands for Attention Deficit Hyperactivity Disorder and was first recognized in 1902 by a British pediatrician named Sir George Still. He described the disorder as "an abnormal defect of moral control" in children. It wasn't until 1936 that the FDA approved a medicine called Benzedrine, manufactured by Smith, Kline and French, the precursor to GlaxoSmithKline. Dr. Charles Bradley gave it to his young patients for respiratory ailments; an unexpected side effect was they performed better in school. Sadly, his findings were not widely accepted. In 1955, Ciba Pharmaceutical Company (now part of Novartis) began marketing Ritalin as a psychostimulant, which ended up being a successful treatment for ADHD. It is still popular today.

In 1980, the DSM III, the third edition of the psychiatry handbook of mental diseases and disorders, published a distinction between ADHD and ADD, which are in essence the same but the latter not including the hyperactivity symptom. By the year 2000, there were three distinctions of the disorder to help target specific treatments.

In 2011, the Center for Disease Control (CDC) reported that 11% of children in America have been diagnosed with ADHD. However, according to the American Psychiatric Association, only 5% actually have ADHD. These two statements literally contradict each other, unless psychiatrists are blindly diagnosing kids to help Big Pharma sell their medications. Also in 2011, 6.1% of America's youth, age 4-17, were taking medication to treat ADHD. The recommended treatment for preschoolers, ages 4-5, is behavioral therapy; however half of the group who were diagnosed were prescribed medication such as Adderall. Simply put, Adderall is a central nervous system stimulant that affects the chemicals in the brain. One of the many side effects is the potential for delayed growth in children and doctors must follow-up frequently with young patients. Adderall is also addictive, suppresses appetite, and can lead to psychosis if misdiagnosed. Giving this to a 5 year old is tantamount to child abuse. To give any kind of mind altering drug to a child who doesn't even have a fully formed brain yet is unnatural, unhealthy, and guaranteed to have long term health repercussions.

As recently as 2013, studies are showing such a dramatic increase in the diagnosis of high school age kids of ADHD, it seems it is being treated as an epidemic. Forbes reported that 15% of high school age kids are currently labeled with ADHD. The truth of the matter is that only about 5% actually have it. Forbes continues in their article:

> "This gross over-diagnosis and prescription is a direct result of intense, multi-million dollar marketing campaigns by the drug makers, both through

celebrity endorsements as well print and television ads that prompt patients and their families to ask doctors about those specific drugs. The result is to sway doctors to go for the easy, quick fix solution of a pill (when you have a hammer, everything you see is a nail). And the tactic has paid off, with a quintupling of stimulant sales since 2002, to over $8 billion in revenues."

ADHD can be managed without medication. While time and patience are needed, children who are not medicated learn how to manage the disorder on their own. When they reach full adulthood, the disorder is a little easier to manage because the part of the brain that controls impulse isn't fully formed until age 19-21.

Dr. Gregory Fabiano published in Clinical Psychology Review in 2009 his results from a meta-analysis that proved behavioral treatment is as or more effective than medication. There are three types of concurrent approaches: parent programs, teacher programs and therapeutic recreational programs. The parent programs are teaching parents how to positively and immediately reinforce good behavior. Teacher programs are designed to modify teaching styles for kids with ADHD. One example he used is a child who hated math, disturbed his classmates, and became a disruption to the class. The teacher began hiding the answer on his worksheets in invisible ink so when he finished a problem, he could reveal the answer right away. Brilliant! The last piece, with the recreational programs can be challenging to keep them running, but worth the effort for the kids who benefit from them. Learning crafts and activities with other kids, consistently focusing on team work and other positive behaviors help kids learn how to manage their disorder. The answer to every problem isn't always a pill.

Another example of Big Pharma's control over society in the name of greed is the diagnosis of social anxiety. It is merely a set of behaviors, proven to be cured with therapeutic treatment, which the pharmaceutical companies and psychiatrists label as a "disease" solely for the purpose of selling drugs. Not all psychiatrists buy into Big Pharma's bullshit, but as mentioned before, sales reps make their mortgage on the number of prescriptions sold.

What exactly is social anxiety disorder? Essentially, it is overpowering anxiety and extreme self-consciousness in social situations. Symptoms include nervousness, shyness, negative thought patterns, and feeling fearful of "screwing up" in front of everyone. It is merely a "medicalization" of normal human behavior. Who hasn't been nervous to speak in front of a group or give a presentation? How about entering a room filled with strangers? Of course people will feel nervous or anxious! Does that necessarily mean they have a disease or need to be medicated? Just another easy way out for people to feel good, not address their emotions and Big Pharma is right there to help them along. Pharmaceutical companies actually market and promote social anxiety in the name of increasing sales of mind altering drugs.

The National Institute of (Mental) Health reported the National Comorbidity Survey-Adolescent Supplement where they interviewed 10,000 youths between the ages of 13 and 18, face to face. They assessed the kids using standard diagnostic criteria set by the American Psychiatric Association's DSM-IV. The results were interesting. 50% of those surveyed categorized themselves as shy. Of those 50%, about 12% met the criteria for social anxiety disorder, approximately 600 kids. Of the other 50% who did not classify themselves as shy, 5% met the criteria for social anxiety disorder. There were no blood tests, urine samples, X-rays, EKG, EEG, nor MRIs done. Just questions asked by NIH professionals and answered by teens. Is this an indicator of how mental disease is diagnosed?

Other effective treatments for social anxiety are Cognitive Behavioral Therapy (CBT), psychoanalytic therapy, as well as changes in diet and adding meditation to your daily routine. CBT helps patients manage their anxiety, guiding them to think rational thoughts when faced with their fears. Because so many anxiety issues are rooted in childhood experiences, psychoanalytic therapy can be very effective in identifying the event and dealing with it to reduce anxiety. A reduction in caffeine intact can also help resolve the symptoms. Whether you have an anxiety disorder or not, meditation is an excellent way to clear the mind and center yourself; leading to a calmer approach to any of life's challenges.

Not all psychiatrists are in the back pocket of Big Pharma. Below are some quotes, courtesy of http://www.cchr.org/, the Citizens Commission on Human Rights, from renowned psychiatrists, speaking out about how Big Pharma created the disease social anxiety disorder solely to reap the rewards.

"While there has been no shortage of alleged biochemical explanations for psychiatric conditions...not one has been proven. Quite the contrary. In every instance where such an imbalance was thought to have been found, it was later proven false." —*Dr. Joseph Glenmullen, Harvard Medical School psychiatrist*

"The theories are held on to not only because there is nothing else to take their place, but also because they are useful in promoting drug treatment." —*Dr. Elliott Valenstein Ph.D., author of* Blaming the Brain

Depression happens to almost everyone at some point in their life. From losing a loved one, losing a job, poor self-esteem or any other number of reasons, depression can be caused by genetics, biological, environmental, or psychological reasons. MRIs show the brain activity in a patient with depression looks different than one without depression. Isolating the parts of the brain that involve mood, sleep, appetite and behavior help doctors understand how depression affects the brain, however it cannot help with diagnosis because it is not clear yet in what ways the chemicals in the brain interact to relieve symptoms.

In America's youth, 3.3% experience depression according to NIH (National Institutes of Health), yet in 2009 the CDC reported that 4.8% of teens were using medications to treat depression, that number rising every year.

Antidepressants function by working with the neurotransmitters in the brain and "balancing" the chemicals called serotonin and norepinephrine. The NIH also states that, "Scientists have found that these particular chemicals are involved in regulating mood, but they are unsure of the exact ways that they work." So even though they do not know exactly how they work, nor do they know long term effects of giving them to our children, 4.8% of them are taking medications anyhow.

The most popular medications are SSRIs, or selective serotonin reuptake inhibitors such as Prozac, Zoloft, Lexapro, Paxil and Celexa. Of the selection of antidepressants available, these have the least amount of side effects, though can still cause nausea, headaches, jitters and insomnia. In teens, it can also lead to suicidal thoughts or even suicide attempts. Older drugs, tricyclics are powerful but extremely dangerous. They can affect people with heart conditions, cause drowsiness and weight gain. MAOIs (monoamine oxidase inhibitors) are the oldest class of antidepressants and though it is effective treatment for atypical depression, the host of side effects is long. There is a long list of foods that must be avoided, as well as complications with other medications such as birth control pills, prescription pain killers, cold and allergy medications and herbal supplements. When MAOIs are mixed with SSRIs, the likelihood of serotonin syndrome increases; symptoms include confusion, hallucinations and seizures. Sound like fun?

A quick look at the top medications that are padding Big Pharma's already overflowing wallet. Cymbalta was the top seller for 2013, adding $4 billion in revenue to Eli Lilly's sales. The patent expired at the end of the year, opening the market up to generic competition, and dropping Lilly's revenues. Eli Lilly also first manufactured the infamous Prozac in 1987, a drug requiring to black label warnings by the FDA about suicide as a side effect, especially in teens. Pristiq, a drug owned by Wyeth, was a distant second in 2013 ringing up $600 million in sales. Because it is a time released drug, and the dosage for effectiveness cannot be reduced, it is a drug that is difficult to stop taking. The drop in mood and mental state when stopping antidepressants "cold turkey" can have horrible side effects, including a return of the depression it once treated.

Like all natural remedies, St. John's Wort (SJW) has borne the brunt of much criticism. It is a plant that has many medicinal uses, and comes in many forms. It can be sipped in tea, taken in pill form, liquid form, and used topically. SJW is an antiseptic and anti-inflammatory, and also has the potential to treat depression. Critics will cite that "recent studies have shown" (vague catchall phrase Big Pharma uses when discrediting competition) that SJW is no more effective than placebos. If that is true, why do Europeans use it extensively to treat mild to moderate depression? In 2000, the FDA issued a warning that SJW may interfere with a plethora of medications, treating a wide range of ailments. Diseases such as heart, depression (SSRIs and MAOIs), seizures and cancer to name a few can have adverse issues when taken with SJW. A study published in Public Health Nutrition took articles and papers written from 1960-2000 on SJW. They combined all the data on them from efficacy, side effects and drug interactions. Their conclusion? SJW is a promising antidepressant that needs more investigation as the data are not sufficient to accept it as a first line treatment for depression.

Big Pharma prevented many studies from getting off the ground because of the inherent competition the potential treatment would cause, and since there is no money to be made on natural supplements, you can bet they want to suppress any and all information on SJW being an effective treatment.

With all of these statistics, drug warnings, and other dangerous side effects, why are we allowing our children to be drugged by Big Pharma? Children who begin taking central nervous system drugs or SSRIs at a young age are usually on them for a significant portion of their youth. How does it affect their development into adulthood? Altering the chemical make-up of a youth can have an effect on their ability to truly know who they are. Imagine being in a mental fog for half of your life, and once the fog is lifted, the confusion and detachment to yourself could be profound. Not to mention, Freud believed sexuality was the key to development. SSRIs affect the sex drive, essentially numbing our ability to get aroused. Does this stunt the development of our children, denying them the ability for human connection? Only time will tell.

In recent years, the anti-vaccination movement has sparked powerful debates among parents and physicians. We have Big Pharma to thank for the debate to have even been started. Ever since the day Edward Jenner, the father of immunology, discovered the smallpox vaccine, there has been controversy surrounding the vaccination of our children. Initially, concerns in 1796 were vastly different than 200 plus year later. The smallpox vaccine was created by the puss from cowpox blisters. Concerns then were sanitation, religious, political and questioning the science behind it. Nowadays, the concerns are how much control Big Pharma has on society, whether or not the vaccines cause autism, and proof the vaccines do not perpetuate the disease.

Because Big Pharma has become this behemoth monster, a multi-billion dollar mysterious conglomerate with shady, back door dealings with physicians and our government, it is ripe for conspiracy theorists who think pharmaceutical companies are trying to poison their children. These parents who feel vaccines do more damage than good are putting all our children at risk for diseases that had literally been wiped off the planet. In the name of protecting their assets and making money through unethical means, they have created a whole subset of society that fears them to the point of endangering children. Without vaccines, diseases like pertussis (whooping cough) are making a comeback and infecting kids all over the country.

But the question is, are the anti-vaxxers right? According to an article published in Rolling Stone magazine by Robert F. Kennedy Jr. in 2005, there is a BIG cover up. The Big Pharma companies knew back in 1991 that the mercury based preservative thimerosal, used in vaccines, causes significant health issues in infants, most critically tied to autism. Instead of immediately alerting physicians, issuing recalls, or taking proper steps to rectify the dire situation, they conspired on how best to cover it up. Why? Because lawsuits could seriously deplete their bottom line.

The CDC paid the Institute of Medicine to conduct another study that down plays the risk of vaccinations containing thimerosal. Politicians aren't innocent either in this mess:

> "The drug companies are also getting help from powerful lawmakers in Washington. Senate Majority Leader Bill Frist, who has received $873,000 in contributions from the pharmaceutical industry, has been working to immunize vaccine makers from liability in 4,200 lawsuits that have been filed by the parents of injured children."
> (http://www.globalresearch.ca/vaccinations-deadly-immunity/14510)

Talk about a conflict of interest! The very men we elect to represent us in Washington, DC are sitting in the back pockets of Big Pharma, helping them protect their bottom line. What is worse, Eli Lilly who first manufactured thimerosal, tested it back in 1930 by injecting 22 patients suffering from terminal meningitis. All 22 died within two weeks of receiving the shot. Yet, Lilly did not disclose with results of this study, nor did it stop them from promoting their vaccine preservative. With the spike in autism in the 1990's in the US, there is an even bigger increase in India and other developing countries, which now use thimerosal-laced vaccines. Is there no stopping Big Pharma?

It is a proven fact that vaccines help inoculate children from deadly, highly contagious diseases. Because the percentage of autistic children who have been vaccinated is low, the risk with immunizations is worth the potential for autism. No parent wants to harm their child, and sometimes the feeling to protect them is overpowering. Saying no to vaccinations opens them up to a whole host of potentially killer viruses. It is irresponsible of the government agencies to not have enough studies to guarantee the safety of vaccines for our children. If they were to conduct enough studies to have viable, concrete facts and allow the drug companies to change their recipes for the vaccines, there would be no argument.

Chapter 5: Conspiracy Theories

With such a long, complicated and often confusing history, filled with mergers and acquisitions, it comes as no surprise that there is no shortage of conspiracy theories tied to Big Pharma. As with any conspiracy, there is always a ring of truth in the story. And even at times, it may be the truth without any evidence available to prove it.

Shelley Belcourt, a former RN turned entrepreneur has a website dedication to helping people market their business online, and her personal passion is kids health, specifically taking a natural approach to medicine. She also has a detailed timeline of how Big Pharma grew into the colossal cartel it is today. Summarized from her website:

> May 15, 1911, the US Supreme Court finds John Rockefeller and his Trust guilty of racketeering and corruption. Technically, the trust was dismantled. By 1913,

Rockefeller planned to take over the pharmaceutical industry, a growing business sector, by using something called "philanthropy" where he was able to hide money in a tax haven allowing him to support and control the pharmaceutical industry. All the money went to medical schools and hospitals; they were the missionaries of the companies who manufactured the new hot products known as synthetic drugs.

In 1918, Rockefeller uses the Spanish flu epidemic to begin a "witch hunt" on any drug marketed on which they didn't already own the patent. In 1925, across the pond in Europe, IG Farben is born and a new cartel begins to gain power. In 1929, the Rockefeller cartel and the IG Farben cartel split the globe into interest spheres, the crime which Rockefeller was found guilty of in 1911.

1932-33, IG Farben doesn't want to be restrained to the agreed upon areas on interest in the globe. They throw their support behind Adolf Hitler, who promises to conquer the world for them militarily. Every country Germany invades, they turned over all chemical, petrochemical and pharmaceutical company over to IG Farben.

1942-45, IG Farben tests its soon to be patented drugs in Auschwitz, Dauchau and other concentrations camps. The fees for these studies went directly from Bayer, Hoechst, and BASF to the SS who controlled the concentration camps. Degesch held the trademark on Zyklon B, the poisonous gas used in extermination camps. It may be shocking to learn that IG Farben owned 42% of Degesch. A total of 24 managers from Bayer, Hoechst and BASF were tried, 13 found guilty of mass murder, leading wars of aggression, and instituting slavery. Fritz Ter Meer, sentenced to 12 years in prison, was released and returned to his role as Chairman of the Board of Bayer.

Back in America in 1944, Nelson Rockefeller was already knee deep in politics as Under-Secretary of the State and later, Special Advisor to President Truman. Rockefeller was keeping the family's interests protected from inside the US government.

Allegedly, Rockefeller assisted in the creation of the United Nations, World Health Organization, and World Trade Organization.

Direct from Belcourt's website, under the heading 1963:

"Under the pretense of consumer protection, it launched a four-decade-long crusade to outlaw vitamin therapies and other natural, non-patentable health approaches in all member countries of the United Nations. The goal was to simply ban any and all competition for the multi-billion dollar business with patented drugs. The plan was simple: copy for the entire world what had already been accomplished in America in the 1920s – a monopoly on health care for the investment business with patented drugs.

Since the marketplace for the pharmaceutical investment business depends upon the continued existence of diseases, the drugs it developed were not intended to prevent, cure or eradicate disease. Thus, the goal of the global strategy was to monopolize health for billions of people, with pills that nearly cover symptoms but hardly ever address the root cause of disease. The deprivation of billions of people from having access to life saving information about the health benefits of natural health approaches,

> whilst at the same time establishing a monopoly with largely ineffective and frequently toxic patented drugs, caused disease and death in genocidal proportions."
> http://shelleybelcourt.com/history-of-the-pharmaceutical-companies/

This alone holds some very big nuggets of truth. If Big Pharma is allowed to continue drugging America, there will be no cures and no end to new diseases. Whether you believe in conspiracy theories or not, this is a persuasive argument that literally hits the nail on the head of what's wrong with health care today.

The US government is elected by the people, for the people. Or at least it is supposed to be. In truth, Big Pharma controls the government and there is a long laundry list of evidence and fines paid to prove it. The pharmaceutical industry is the third largest contributor of funds to election campaigns. Perhaps they learned that from IG Farben who managed to fund Hitler's regime. In the 2011-2012 election year, Big Pharma and friends contributed over $10 million to various campaigns. Often, the quantity of cash increases in election years where new initiatives are on the table. Case in point, when Medicare Part D was under debate in 2002 and the Affordable Care Act was being finalized in 2008, contributions spiked.

OpenSecret.org is a website dedicated to tracking and reporting corporate contributions amounts and compiling statistics. In 2013-2014, Pfizer was the number one pharmaceutical company to contribute to elections campaign, totaling over $1.5 million. The top recipients of these funds were Mitch McConnell (R-KY) with over $359,000 in donations and Ed Markey (D-MA) bringing in $305,000. Campaign contributions are a legal form of influencing the law makers to protect the interests of the corporations who donate. The bigger the corporation, the bigger the donation nets the most power.

In April of 2014, the Supreme Court ruled to eliminate a long standing cap on donation amounts by an individual to candidates in a two year election cycle. The ruling passed 5-4, and the four that were against it were vehemently opposed to it. Though they admittedly said the prosecutors did an excellent job presenting their case, Justice Stephen G. Breyer, who was against the ruling commented now that the cap was eliminated, "a single individual can contribute millions of dollars to a political party or to a candidate's campaign." Since it is illegal for corporations to make donations unless under the umbrella of a PAC (Political Action Committee), Big Pharma makes the contributions on an individual level. With the elimination of the cap for individuals, pharmaceutical companies can keep lining the pockets of politicians to keep protecting their interests, and letting them get away with murder, figuratively and literally.

The power of Big Pharma continues to gain and grow, even when they admittedly break the law.

CNN reported in 2010 the Pfizer scandal involving Bextra, a drug that was approved by the FDA in 2001. It was only approved as a treatment for arthritis and menstrual cramps, yet sales reps illegally promoted it as a painkiller for surgeries, prescribed in higher doses for which it was approved. The FDA had safety concerns about using it for this purpose as it has been linked to heart attacks and strokes. Not to mention it was $3 per pill as opposed to pennies for ibuprofen or Tylenol for post-surgical pain. A former sales rep for Pfizer turned whistle blower, Glenn DeMott, when asked if the sales reps knew what they were doing was illegal, answered "...the district manager approved it saying it might not be legal but if they don't make their numbers, they are not going to keep their job." Mike Loucks, a former federal prosecutor commented that pushing a drug illegally makes a mockery of the FDA.

Pfizer was faced with a very serious charge, because if any pharmaceutical company is found guilty of fraud, they are immediately removed from the Medicare and Medicaid programs. Losing the income from these programs is the death knell for any corporations. They would be out of business, which means thousands of people out of jobs, and millions of people without medication. Yet how is Pfizer still doing business?

Pfizer owns a subsidiary called Pharmacia Corp, which owns a subsidiary named Pharmacia and Upjohn LLC, and they own another subsidiary called Pharmacia and Upjohn Company, who in turn owns Pharmacia and Upjohn Company Inc. Confusing? It's supposed to be. Visually it looks like this:

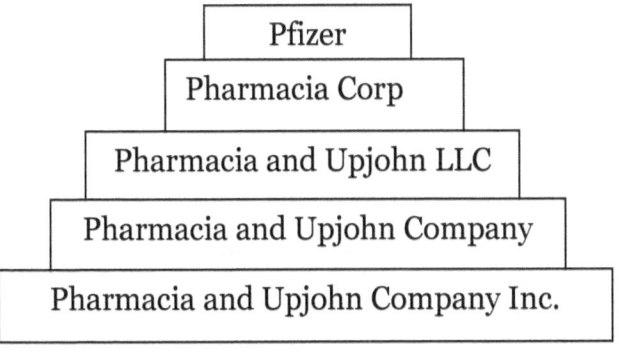

Pfizer is the parent company of all four of the subsidiaries. What does Pharmacia and Upjohn Company Inc. sell? Nothing. It is a shell company created by Pfizer in March of 2007 for the sole purpose that if they got caught in an illegal act, they had a company to take the fall for them. The feds, knowing what potential harm could come to the economy and patients who rely on Pfizer continuing to conduct business, made a deal with Pfizer. They were fined $1.3 billion for the illegal act, paid another $1 billion in civil suits, and their shell company, Pharmacia and Upjohn Company Inc. was kicked out of Medicare and Medicaid. The $2.3 billion total paid out was chalked up to the cost of doing business. In reality, it only represented three months' worth of profit. The Department of Health and Human Services enforced an integrity agreement, which required those in charge to sign a document stating they will not conduct business illegally, and included that they install a tracking program that monitors sales reps and the prescriptions sold in their territories. By doing this, it will allow Pfizer to red flag any suspicious trends in prescription medications. Does the punishment fit the crime? What can we do to keep Big Pharma honest?

According to www.fda.gov, in June of 1906, President Theodore Roosevelt signed into law the Pure Food and Drug Act, also known as the Wiley Act, named for Harvey Washington Wiley who was chief chemist for the Bureau of Chemistry, a division of the Department of Agriculture, the FDA's predecessor. Wiley was dedicated to researching the adulteration and misbranding of products, such as pharmaceuticals, in the American market. He lobbied for a law to be passed that would create a universal standard for all consumables to be marketed and sold in America. The main function of the FDA then and today is to act as a federal consumer protection agency.

The responsibilities of the FDA include:

- Protecting the public health by assuring the safety, effectiveness, quality, and security of human and veterinary drugs, vaccines and other biological products, and medical devices. The FDA is also responsible for the safety and security of most of our nation's food supply, all cosmetics, dietary supplements and products that give off radiation.
- Regulating tobacco products.

In order for a drug to be certified by the FDA, it must go through extensive testing beginning with laboratory and animal testing. Once sufficient information has been gathered, the next stage is testing on humans, ensuring it is safe and effective for diagnostics or treatment for which it was intended. Once the testing is complete, the drug company must fill out an NDA or New Drug Application. The application includes all the findings from the testing, details on proper manufacturing to ensure the company can actually produce the drug, and lastly a proposed label that includes uses, dosage, and other vital information for the patients purchasing the drug.

The FDA has not always been as honest as its roots. Wiley's vision has been tainted by greed over the decades, and in 1999 the FDA approved a drug that would become the center of one of the biggest drug scandals in history. Vioxx, manufactured by Merck was promoted as a painkiller, NSAID (non-steroid anti-inflammatory drug) which was gentle on the digestive track. Within a short period of the drug being released on the market, reportedly there were 80 million patients taking the medication. In 2001, the FDA approved a label change, declaring it safer on the stomach than its competitor, leading to more sales for Merck. In 2003, a study Merck conducted showed a 39% increase in risk of heart attack within the first 90 days of taking the medication over patients taking Celebrex, its direct competitor. It wasn't withdrawn from the market until 2004. The result of the collaboration between the FDA and Merck led to over 55,000 deaths. In 2007, Merck settled a class action suit for a whopping $4.85 billion. The FDA apologized for its "lack of effective oversight and promised to do better in the future." (http://readersupportednews.org/)

In response to the Vioxx scandal, the FDA created the Transparency Initiative in 2009. This was established to help Americans feel better informed of the processes and decisions the FDA makes. The initiative states on www.fda.gov:

Summary of Phase III: Transparency to Regulated Industry

> In January 2011, the Transparency Task Force released a report describing 19 action items FDA is implementing to improve its transparency to regulated industry. The report also proposed 5 additional draft proposals for public comment.FDA accepted

public comment on the proposals on this website from January 6, 2011 through March 6, 2011.

Summary of Tasks: Draft Proposals for Public Comment

The action items and draft proposals for public comment fall under five broad topic areas:

- Communicating Information about Agency Procedures
- Product Application Review Process
- Guidance Development
- Regulations Development
- Import Process

Wonderful news for Americans, right? Sadly, the FDA is still right in the back pocket of Big Pharma. While these transparency initiatives seem like a big step in the right direction, merely 11 months after the policy began implementation, the FDA gathered medical experts for a committee to determine if the dangers of drospirnone outweigh the benefits of the drug.

Drospirenone is the active ingredient in Bayer's birth control pills, Yaz and Yasmin. Women who take this drug are seven times more likely to have a thromboembolism, which is a fancy name for a blood clot that can lead to heart attacks, stroke, and yes, even death. Yaz and Yasmin were the hottest birth control pills on the market, raking in money for Bayer.

The committee voted to keep the drug on the shelves by a four vote margin. Four of the panelists on the committee had financial ties to Bayer, either previously working for them, licensees, or received research funds. The FDA opted not to disclose this information. So much for transparency! Ironically, the FDA had barred a panelist, Dr. Sidney Wolfe, before the committee began, because of an intellectual conflict of interest as he advised his readers not to take Yaz because of the limited data available.

The FDA continues to talk out of both sides of its mouth. They tell the American people they are going to be more forthcoming with information, to "help" citizens by providing the necessary information they need to make well-informed decisions. Yet, they collude with Big Pharma to protect their resources. The moral of the story? Greed is dangerous.

To complete the trinity of the "Medical Mafia", the American Medical Association was created in 1847 by Dr. Nathan Davis. The goal of the AMA was and still is to promote the art and science of medicine and the betterment of public health. The AMA has a long history of doing good, however since the 1920's, when it began policing every surgical practice and general health methodology, the do good part became tainted. This is around the time Rockefeller began his involvement in "philanthropy" and as the mafia grew, the three in control were the FDA, Big Pharma (Rockefeller's cartel), and the AMA. If it wasn't a practice approved of by the FDA and Big

Pharma, the AMA acted as enforcer to suppress, discredit and stop alternative medical practices.

This came to a head in the early 1950's when Congressman Charles Tobey recruited Benedict Fitzgerald, an investigator for the Interstate Commerce Commission to look into allegations of conspiracy and monopolistic activity in "orthodox" medicine, i.e. the AMA. The reason Tobey recruited Fitzgerald is his son, Tobey Jr. was diagnosed with cancer and given 2 years to live. Tobey sought all potential treatments, and chose an alternative one not promoted by the AMA. His son was cured. Tobey couldn't fathom why these practices were not more widely known and available to the public. In what became known as The Fitzgerald Congressional Report of 1953, Fitzgerald states:

"My investigation to date should convince this committee that a conspiracy does exist to stop the free flow and use of drugs in interstate commerce which allegedly has solid therapeutic value. Public and private funds have been thrown around like confetti at a country fair to close up and destroy clinics, hospitals, and scientific research laboratories which do not conform to the viewpoint of medical associations." - Benedict F. Fitzgerald, Jr., Special Counsel, US Senate Committee on Interstate and Foreign Commerce, 1953

The AMA has been tethered to the pharmaceutical industry for decades. Why would an organization who promotes "the betterment of public health" have a long history of opposing public health reform? The AMA has lobbied against health care reform included in the New Deal in 1933, the inception of Medicare, and blocked health reform in 1993. The answer should be obvious at this point. It all comes down to money.

Chapter 6: Squelching Innovative Medical Practices

Natural remedies or homeopathy was discovered in the late 18th century by German physician Samuel Hahnemann. He was known for his work in a wide range of area including pharmacology. His breakthrough discovery on how homeopathic remedies work was during an experiment with cinchon, a Peruvian bark that supposedly cures malaria. Back then, there were no formal laboratories, research teams and committees per se, so he tested the theory on himself. Soon after he began his experiment, he presented with symptoms of malaria such as high fever. Those same symptoms went away when he stopped taking the cinchon. Because of his work, we now know the following rules to be true:

> Like cures like: By consuming small, even trace amounts of what has infected you; it spurs the body into fighting off the ailment with antibodies produced in the

immune system. The small amount of like substance trains your immune system for battle with the real deal.

The more diluted the remedy, the more powerful: Hahnemann continued diluting the substance to get it below toxic levels. By doing so, it made the remedy more potent. This has lent fuel for critics saying homeopathic remedies that are tested by traditional scientists contain nothing but water and alcohol. Today, science still has not explained this fully however the answer is in quantum physics and the emerging field of energy medicine. A Harvard study using a nuclear electromagnetic resonance test concluded that there were distinct readings of subatomic activity in 23 homeopathic remedies. Somehow, through dilution and succession (shaking of the remedy), an electromagnetic frequency is somehow imprinted in the solution. Remember Rife and his cancer cure?

Illness is specific to the individual: This is pretty self-explanatory, considering no two people are exactly alike (except identical twins). Everyone has unique DNA, and symptoms affect people differently. Certainly some of the same medications help some of the same people however, homeopathy takes a customized approach to treating the patient.

Since herbs and other natural substances found in nature cannot be patented, Big Pharma ensures laws are made to keep holistic remedies buried. With deep pockets and power within the media and government, they use the FDA to support their findings and the AMA to enforce traditional, conventional medicine. Not only do they suppress public knowledge about homeopathy, they out and out discredit anyone and any company that supports holistic healing and natural methods.

In the 1970's, Dr. John A. Richardson piloted trials on the effectiveness of B17 in curing cancer. He prescribed the patients vitamin B17, a vegetarian diet, and other vitamins minerals for a fully balanced approach. He not only cured patients, but they went on to live long and healthy lives. He was eventually arrested and stripped of his medical license for his findings, and it is illegal to treat cancer with vitamin B17 in the United States.

Rene Caisse, a nurse in Toronto, Canada came across an old Native American recipe for a tea containing burdock root, slippery elm inner bark, sheep sorrel, and Indian rhubarb root. All of these plants are indigenous to Canada. She produced the tea for her aunt, diagnosed with terminal cancer. Her aunt's doctor, R.O. Fisher supervised the treatment. Her aunt not only was cured of cancer, but lived for another 21 years. Sadly, there is not much data on Essaic because of the suppression of the Big Pharma cartels. The tea is still available through the internet, but be wary of counterfeits. It must be the trademarked version, made in Canada.

As with most homeopathic treatments, there is little to no information about their complete effectiveness, nor any clinical trials that can support the initial claims of the pioneers, or their patients. What can be gleaned from this, just as conventional medicine leaders say, cancer won't be cured with just one drug, it will take a cocktail. Wouldn't it be more effective to try a combination of homeopathic and synthetic medicines? Big Pharma disagrees, because their bottom line will suffer.

Chapter 7: Helpless in America

As Americans living in the land of the free and home of the brave, it is our duty to our families and each other to stop Big Pharma and the Medical Mafia. While it may not happen overnight, it can certainly happen if we stop drugging ourselves to the point of becoming passive sheep that blindly follow what the trusted doctors, pharmaceutical companies, FDA, and AMA tell us. We must take action to break the bonds that tie Big Pharma to our government and its agencies. Stop feeding the greed that has become so great and powerful within Big Pharma, they have too much control over our lives.

One action that every American should take is to become educated. Upon researching this book, it required checking and cross-checking facts for hours on end. However, it is imperative that every American who goes to the doctor and is prescribed a medication to know the details of their doctor, i.e. what pharmaceutical companies do they have ties with? Have they received kickbacks for the medication they are prescribing you? And more importantly, what does the drug do to help your condition? What are the side effects? It is equally important to ask about alternative medicine. What other options are available to you?

Americans are caught in a crux between being too busy to care and too passive to do anything about it. The expectation we all have is when we are ill or not feeling well, we go to the doctor and get medication. We take the medication, we feel better, and we pick up our lives where we left off. STOP BEING SUCH SHEEP, AMERICA! Wake up! Your email can wait five minutes while you read up on what you are taking.

Another powerful tool right at the fingertips of Americans is social media. Facebook, Twitter, Instagram, SnapChat, and countless others are available for you to spread the word and get people interested in paying attention. Discuss what your doctor prescribes and for what with your friends and family, let people know because it takes just one person to read it and say, "hey, me too!" and before you know it, the information has gone viral.

Social media has the power to make or break a story. If used responsibly and with proper knowledge, awareness about the Big Pharma cartel can spread like wildfire.

When doing research on drugs, ensure you are getting data from the clinical trials and not a promotional website. Everything gets skewed on the internet, and the truth is out there, you just have to dig a little. It is important to even question clinical trials. With the effectiveness of search engine optimization, most articles have embedded links to other studies – click on them! There is no such thing as having too much information. Think of the research as garnering battle gear. Every little piece you gather is another piece of armor with which you can go out into the world. Make sure the statistics make sense, and then go search the same data out from another source. Getting conflicting information? Welcome to the Age of the Internet. Keep digging!

It is critical for us, as responsible citizens, to not point fingers at Big Pharma without the armor to fight a battle with them. If you feel the drug doctors have prescribed for you, your children, your spouse or parents is not right, and you don't want to risk the side effects? Make sure you know everything you can before taking it to your doctor or social media.

Drugs in America cost significantly more than in Europe. For example, Nexium which is used to treat acid reflux, costs about $30 in France. Here in America, it is $187. Why? Because Big Pharma is raping Americans hard earned money. A website called truthout.org has suggested a plan. The reason we don't have the buying power here in America is because we don't have a single payer health program. Well, technically we do, and it's called Medicare Part D. Only problem is it is strictly for the elderly, and Congress made sure to add a piece of legislature into it declaring that all participants will pay full price. The Veterans Administration receives a 40% discount on all prescription drug costs because of their massive buying power. If the Medicare Part D were for everyone, ages 0 and up, the buying power of the average American citizen would be huge. Drop the clause about paying full price under the act, and pow! You have a single payer healthcare program for every citizen, with negotiating power to reduce the cost of drugs. Support this act by writing to your congressman.

The worst thing we can do is stay the course we are on. Blindly taking whatever medication our doctor prescribes, without so much as a question as to why. The definition of insanity is to continue doing the same thing and expecting different outcomes. We cannot continue doing the same thing and expect Big Pharma to change. It won't without a fight; that is a guarantee.

Conclusion

The purpose of this book is not to turn you away from conventional medicine, nor to think that Big Pharma and Big Brother are watching your every move. The goal is to create an awareness; one that will stick with you for your long life. This book has pulled from many, many resources to help the American people open their eyes and come out of the drugged sleep in which Big Pharma has placed us. Certainly, there are people who need medications, mostly the elderly and true psychiatric patients. That group does not make up the 70% of America taking prescription drugs.

As in every aspect of America's existence, we can learn from history. Looking at how Big Pharma started, grew, and gained power into the biggest monopoly in the world can help us understand how we can take them down. They are built on money; sales in the billions of dollars. It's our money, America! Stop giving them more power!

A story that correlates with the power that the American people can have on corporate America begins in a town in Massachusetts called Tewksbury. The headquarters for a supermarket chain called Market Basket is located there. Market Basket is one of the largest, and certainly most profitable supermarkets in New England. The business is family owned and run since 1917, when two Greek immigrants opened a grocery store in Lowell, MA specializing in lamb. The chain grew into 75 strong stores, and handed down two generations of Demoulas sons. They are most well-known for their great value and variety of product as well as how much the employees love working there. All the upper management began as bag boys and cashiers. It is not unheard of for cashiers to have worked for 10 or more years with the company, for their profit sharing is second to none. The family squabbled through the years, lawsuits and inheritances fought over. From 1990-2014 saw the bitterest fight to date.

On July 18, 2014, the Board of Directors fired the president of the company, the grandson of the original owners. The cousin who was involved in shifting the power in the board wanted to sell the company and collect his portion. Interestingly enough, the former president, named Arthur T. Demoulas, didn't really care about the money, he was distraught as to what would happen to the company, its employees and the community. To show how beloved the president was, all the employees protested outside the stores with signs like "Artie T is Our President" and "Reinstate Artie T". They weren't after better benefits or higher pay because they already had it! They wanted their president back. The community, knowing full well the family history, and how loved Artie T was by the employees also protested. The citizens voted with their wallet. Stores that were normally packed on Saturdays were empty of customers. This is a company that earned $4 billion in revenue a year. All seventy-five stores were devoid of customers for almost 8 weeks. After protests, bans, many letters, even politicians quoted they wanted to see Artie T back in the presidency, the Board of Directors reached an agreement whereby Artie T would buy his cousin out and own the company outright. On August 27, he was reinstated as president. Business returned to normal by the weekend.

Now this may not be Big Pharma, and even more so than pharmaceuticals, food is a necessity. People shopped elsewhere for the 8 weeks. There are other options for most people who need prescription drugs. Vote with your wallet and watch how fast Big Pharma deflates.

The list of people who are in need of medications to sustain a standard of living is a very short one. For example, take a patient who clearly has a mental disorder such as schizophrenia. There is a need for medication to maintain a normal life, and to perform daily functions. People with Type II diabetes need insulin until there can be enough studies done on alternative medicine to prevent or even cure it. Looking at the very long list of medications most commonly prescribed to the elderly, if Big Pharma were to invest in alternative methods, or at least not discredit those who do; many elderly could be better off with a balance of medication and homeopathic remedies.

How much of the blame can be placed on America? Being bombarded every day with advertisements, Big Pharma spares no expense on their marketing and advertising. Are we the proverbial frog in the pot of water that slowly begins to boil? It is up to us to get out of the pot. To do this, we need to be educated. We need to conduct our own research, go to the source of the studies and look at the larger body of evidence like who paid for this study?

There are plenty of independent researchers out there, like LEF (Life Extension Foundation) who are dedicated to publishing the truth. While the government agencies are colluding with Big Pharma, and even the politicians we elect are guilty, it falls to the American people to become whistle-blowers.

Pro-Pharma supporters say the reason there have been no cures yet for major diseases such as diabetes and Alzheimer's is because of a lack of intellectual progression. Breakthroughs happen all the time, but science needs to progress further before we can find a cure. The reason we haven't found a cure is because we have not explored all avenues of treatment, only the ones that earn Big Pharma the most money.

The drugging of our youth is a disgrace and should be penalized under the law. When this stoned generation ages and the true effects of what these drugs have done to their minds becomes apparent, will it be time to hold Big Pharma accountable then? Almost all children are hyper and active, and small percentages do have true ADHD or ADD. However, these mental disorders can be managed with additional care from parents, teachers, and other extracurricular activities. Every teen has felt depressed, unloved, and has said things they don't mean. The majority of the time it is a call for attention, in some cases it is more serious and may require some form of treatment. Sadly, the answer most often provided is prescribing them drugs.

Conspiracy theories will always be abounding in any industry or business that does not conduct transparent affairs. The FDA who committed to a transparency policy clearly didn't respect the policy, thereby creating even more fodder for conspiracy theorists. Every theory has a note of truth in it, and all the scandals such as Bextra and Vioxx contribute to the veracity of the theories. The bottom line truth is that Big Pharma needs to be reined in and the monopoly broken up. Alternative treatments need to be studied, verified and marketed as equally as conventional medicine, regardless of the profit loss to Big Pharma.

Scandals, fraud, bribery and lies... no, this is not a description for the hottest new movie out of

Hollywood. This is what Big Pharma has become, and is no better than the Mexican Juarez cartel. They use seductive and misleading marketing techniques to keep America drugged and sedated, allowing them to maintain their monopoly. Stand up and be heard, America. This is our country and it is high time we take it back from Big Pharma.

www.ingramcontent.com/pod-product-compliance
Lightning Source LLC
Chambersburg PA
CBHW030842180526
45163CB00004B/1429